CDT 2023

Den Ken

Current dental Terminology

Current Dental Terminology (CDT) is a code set with illustrative terms created and refreshed by the American Dental Affiliation (ADA) for revealing dental administrations and systems to dental advantages plans.

CDT codes are fundamental for both charging and to report your dental consideration. Without a doubt, you could definitely realize that CDT represents Current Dental Phrasing. In any case, you want a more profound clarification of how to utilize CDT codes in your training.

All things considered, when you work in a dental office, you'll utilize CDT codes in your day to day existence on the off chance that you're taking care of protection claims.

Understanding dental wording is significant for precise dental charging in light of the fact that it can influence your case exactness and income. One of the difficulties is staying up with the latest while rules in regards to those terms change continually.

At Dental Claim Support, we generally stress the significance of instruction among our far off billers. At the point when dental groups move to us, we believe they should feel certain that genuine dental charging specialists are attempting to get their protection claims repaid. Furthermore, with regards to dental charging training, CDT codes are a tremendous subject.

CDT codes can create turmoil because of the perplexing idea of what it is and the way things are utilized while recording a case. It's pivotal to comprehend CDT codes and their motivation since they will influence the rate at which your cases are paid by protection. Legitimate CDT coding will likewise guarantee consistence that will forestall deceitful case accommodation.

In this article, we'll make sense of what CDT is, what to do when it updates, and why it's so essential to comprehend CDT codes and archive them appropriately.

Anyway, what are CDT codes?

Current dental phrasing (CDT) is a bunch of codes with enlightening terms created and refreshed every year by the American Dental Affiliation (ADA). Your group should follow these updates. We will remember ways to stay aware of CDT changes later in this article.

The CDT Code is the authority reference for terms that should be utilized in cases to outsider payers like insurance agency. So how about we separate it as essential as could be expected.

Each code starts with the letter "D" for Dentistry and is trailed by four numbers. The first number will set the code reach or administration type.

Consider it naming a dental methodology with a number.

Here is an illustration of CDT code documentation for a defensive rebuilding:

D2940 defensive rebuilding

Direct position of a helpful material to safeguard tooth or potentially tissue structure. This technique might be utilized to assuage torment, advance mending, or forestall further weakening. Not to be utilized for endodontic access conclusion, or as a base or liner under reclamation.

There are nine primary help code type goes that your dental group should comprehend, and there are around 20-30 normal CDT codes that a regular practice utilizes day to day. Remembering the D0 to D9 reaches will make it more straightforward to track down a code.

Your dental group utilizes these codes to report the administrations your dental specialist has performed for patients. It's a piece of the riddle of appropriately recording a technique.

Utilizing CDT codes on a dental protection guarantee

You want to appropriately record CDT codes to get repayment from protection on a case. Protection denies guarantees that need, or have incorrect CDT coding appended. You can expand your dental practice's income when there is exact CDT coding on a case. To this end understanding CDT is vital.

On the off chance that you submit dental cases as one or the other an in-network or out-of-network dental consideration supplier, your work falls under the HIPAA rules - you need to utilize these codes.

They may currently be available in your dental practice programming, yet you actually need to know how to accurately pick and use them. What's more, this is where seeing each code and the "why" behind CDT coding proves to be useful.

The simplest method for finding the CDT code for a strategy that isn't generally utilized is to decide the technique type range code falls under and search that reach in your training the board programming. This is, obviously just appropriate assuming that you're training the board programming has all of the CDT codes recorded and refreshed inside it.

Utilizing the legitimate code will assist you with keeping away from postpones in guarantee installment, yet it will likewise make less disarray with the patient and insurance agency.

Contingent upon your installment structure, (for the most part material on the off chance that yours is a charge for-administration practice) on the off chance that your patient is anticipating repayment from protection, and this installment is deferred because of erroneous coding - you will probably have an irritated patient.

Yet, inappropriate coding can be a typical error in the event that you're not keeping awake to date on CDT changes, so how might you keep up?

Staying aware of yearly CDT changes to stay consistent

CDT codes are evaluated and refreshed yearly because of innovation and strategies for methods ceaselessly evolving. Not staying aware of these progressions can prompt a couple of issues.

We referenced over that you could confront defers in guarantee repayment; however you could likewise be unintentionally submitting ill-conceived claims that can prompt protection reviews. Regardless of whether it's essentially a misstep - it doesn't make any difference. You would rather not cause your dental practice problems.

CDT updates to search for each year would incorporate the erasure of codes, publication amendments, and new codes being added.

You should make these updates in your training the board programming physically.

For instance, when the new CDT has an erased code, the most ideal way to deal with it in your training the executives programming is to inactivate the code and adhere to your product program guidelines on the best way to refresh your rundown of CDT codes. Try not to erase the erased codes.

In the event that there is another CDT code added, the most ideal way to deal with it is to add the code into your product and arrange it fittingly.

We suggest making a CDT agenda when the yearly updates carry out. We'll share a couple of our specialists' agenda things:

Spending plan for your yearly refreshed CDT coding book

Put resources into a group (clinical and managerial) preparing on the CDT code changes influencing the training

Update the progressions in the Training The board Programming

For a more point by point CDT changes agenda, sign up for our CDT course at Dental Cases Institute - you could procure CE credit.

Fabricate a useful, consistent charging process by putting resources into quality preparation

CDT codes can be a hard subject for dental groups to find out about. Be that as it may, getting ideal case repayment and staying consistent merits the work it takes to find out about CDT. It doesn't need to be a colossal, convoluted secret - you can decide to put resources into your group charging instruction. This decision can prompt a better dental practice - monetarily, by and by, and lawfully.

Dental Cases Institute is an incredible asset for dental groups to find out about CDT coding and different pieces of the dental charging process. This information can prompt more pay for your dental practice, more sure workers, and additional confiding in patients.

What is dental charging? A comprehension of how dental charging functions

At the point when you consider dental charging, as a dental specialist or office chief, you could think "goodness that is our situation to gather cash!" You're correct, and it's more than that. The soundness of your charging framework will represent the moment of truth your dental practice, and understanding the dental charging process is the manner by which you improve and keep up with that wellbeing.

Essentially believing charging is going alright is to gamble with your future. No dental specialist ought to need to experience low assortments since they failed to see how their dental charging framework ought to work. This is what to be aware of dental charging, with extraordinary assistance to comprehend dental protection charging.

On the off chance that you need a sound practice, dental experts really should plainly comprehend how dental charging functions.

Dental Claim Support has been working beginning around 2012 to comprehend, smooth out, and upgrade the dental charging process for dental workplaces. Through this experience as a dental charging organization, we see that numerous dental groups don't grasp the straightforward inquiry of the way this functions.

In this article, we will walk you through a reasonable image of how dental charging functions. It appears to be straightforward, yet figuring out the way this functions and what it involves will assist your dental group with enhancing it such that will acquire additional income from the two patients and dental protection claims. We will respond to the accompanying inquiries:

What is dental charging?

What is the dental charging process?

What is dental charging coding?

What is dental clinical charging?

Is dental charging troublesome?

We will likewise give you a couple of dental charging tips to stick in your back pocket. These are ordinarily posed inquiries that will help your group bill and gather unhesitatingly at your dental practice.

What is dental charging?

Dental charging is any action that gathers installment for dental administrations acted in your dental practice.

What is the dental charging process?

The dental charging process alludes to every one of the means required to get installment from insurance agency and patients for administrations your training gives. The dental charging interaction might be separated into patient charging and protection claims handling - the two fundamental income streams for your training.

Like any cycle, there are clear advances you can follow to travel through the dental charging process effortlessly.

Here is a short agenda of steps in the dental charging process:

1. Gathering patient data - This is finished during the underlying call with the patient when they call to plan their dental arrangement. This data will

incorporate their name, telephone number, address, email address, contract inclinations, and date of birth, name of the endorser's manager or protection plan, protection transporter, transporter's supplier telephone number, protection ID number.

2. Confirming patient protection inclusion - Whenever you've gathered the patient's private and protection data, you'll check it by either calling the insurance agency or signing into your protection gateway. This will provide you with a full breakdown of their advantages that will tell you the condition of their inclusion.

3. Recording dental treatment and code information - As the patient gets treatment the day of their arrangement, somebody in the consideration group keeps the important subtleties in your clinical notes, and codes the systems performed. Typically, an administrator colleague guarantees this is archived, assessed, and electronically endorsed by the supplier in your

dental programming. An everyday approve the day sheet is a best practice to constantly confirm that what occurred in the dental seat is recorded into your product and on your patient's record to be charged.

4. Submitting and following cases and any connections - With the data you've kept in your product, you will currently make, bunch, and present your protection claims. The case will incorporate the code or codes of the technique played out, the patient's all's private and protection data and any connections required. Connections incorporate clinical notes, x-beams, periodontal outlines, stories, essential Eob's, intraoral photographs, and so forth.

5. Settling issues on exceptional cases - In the event that a case has been denied, or 30 days have passed and the case has not been repaid, you should circle back to it. This is called working the protection maturing report. Your biller gets a

rundown of remarkable cases, contacts the insurance agency and sorts out how the case veered off-track, then, at that point, attempts to pursue it for repayment. Here the biller's mastery and effectiveness decide if you see a high assortment rate or a low rate and high above.

6. Charging patients - Contingent upon the income model you've picked, you either charge the patient for the whole measure of the system front and center (expense for administration) or you bill patients the equilibrium subsequent to taking away what their protection advantages ought to cover (repayment model). Patient charging permits you to gather the patient's piece before they leave the dental office or solicitation installment later via mail or email. You then record the case to be repaid by their protection. One way or another, completely gathering on tolerant records receivable is significant on the grounds that it can achieve in around 50% of your income.

7. Posting installments - When your protection guarantee has been paid and saved into your ledger, you'll have to present the installment on your training the executives programming. Doing so keeps all of your data appropriately archived and announced. It likewise finishes the life-pattern of a case and you will actually want to finish it off. Patient installments additionally should be posted expeditiously so your patient bills and income numbers are exact.

8. Running key reports, for example, assortments and record maturing reports - When the installments are posted and the case is finished off, you're ready to truly investigate how your charging exercises are performing to check how well they are gathering installment for what your training produces. Through your dental programming you can run both net creation and net assortment reports as well as remarkable record and protection maturing reports will show you a rundown of

extraordinary cases or potentially tolerant equilibriums that need consideration.

Presently you have an outline that provides you with a thought of what the dental charging process resembles. You can see the lifecycle of a case beginning to end. Understanding this can assist you with remaining focused with how you gather your patient and protection data, and how you work to get your training paid through protection cases and patient installments.

What is dental coding?

Dental coding is the act of utilizing official CDT and additionally ICD-10-CM methodology codes to report conditions and medicines your consideration group performs. These codes are expected for guarantee repayment to remain HIPAA consistent. What you don't know can hurt you: When you inappropriately or incorrectly code a technique, you could unexpectedly commit extortion.

Two code sets most frequently utilized in dental charging are: CDT and ICD-10-CM.

CDT: Current Dental Wording

CDT codes are involved while detailing and reporting dental treatment for a patient. At the end of the day, for any method performed on a patient, there is a particular CDT code that relates to that system. The ongoing year's CDT code set is the authority reference for terms that should be utilized in cases to outsider payers like insurance agency.

These codes start with the letter "D" trailed by 4 numbers.

Here is an illustration of a CDT code:

D2940 defensive rebuilding

Direct position of a supportive material to safeguard tooth as well as tissue structure. This methodology might be utilized to assuage torment, advance recuperating, or forestall further disintegration. Not to be utilized for endodontic access conclusion, or as a base or liner under a rebuilding.

CDT codes are investigated and refreshed yearly. In this manner, you and your group really must keep awake to date on all changes to guarantee the legitimate usage for consistence as well as to guarantee you are getting appropriate repayment.

On the off chance that you submit dental cases as one or the other an in-network or out-of-network dental consideration supplier, or your work falls under HIPAA, you need to utilize these codes. They may currently be available in your dental practice programming, yet you actually need to know how to accurately pick and use them.

ICD-10-CM: Inner Characterization of Infections, 10th Correction, Clinical Adjustment

Like CDT codes, ICD-10-CM is codes used to record and report methodology that are performed by dental specialists, yet clinical in nature. The thing that matters is that the CMS (Habitats for Government health care and Medicaid Administrations) is liable for refreshing the ICD-10-CM yearly. In this way, on account of a dental office, it is utilized when you are documenting a clinical protection guarantee.

ICD-10-CM is additionally refreshed yearly, yet rather than each year starting on January first as CDT are refreshed, ICD-10-CM determined codes become successful starting to have dates of administration on October 1 of each schedule year.

Here are a few instances of how you would record ICD-10-CM codes as it connects with rest apnea or wheezing:

G47.33 Obstructive rest apnea (grown-up) (pediatric)

G47.8 Other rest problems

J98.8 Other indicated respiratory problems

R06.83 Wheezing

ICD-10-CM conveys to the dental and clinical payer data about a patient's dental or clinical condition(s) requiring the treatment recorded on the case structure. Clinical payers expect no less than one conclusion code on the clinical case structure, which is where this code list becomes possibly the most important factor.

Dental coding is significant in the charging system in light of the fact that these codes are utilized to record claims. Insurance agency utilizes the CDT and clinical codes as a premise to repay you for administrations through your protection claims. What's more, it's vital to comprehend codes accurately on the grounds that tolerant installment while utilizing wrong codes can be viewed as misrepresentation, regardless of whether it occurs unintentionally.

What is dental clinical charging?

Dental clinical charging alludes to the most common way of charging clinical protection for care gave in your dental practice.

Now and again the dental specialist performs therapies that fall under the class of clinical consideration. For instance, a dental specialist might treat harmed teeth, gums, and jaw because of mishaps or injury, which is viewed as clinical consideration. A biopsy is another normal clinical treatment dental specialists can perform.

Protection cases ought to go to the clinical protection transporter as essential rather than dental protection, and that is something dental billers need to be aware.

As we referenced above, you are probably going to utilize ICD-10-CM codes while managing methodology that are clinical in nature.

How would you charge clinical protection for dental treatment?

The cycle for recording a dental case and a clinical case has a couple of contrasts.

A clinical case is finished on CMS 1500 structure while a dental case is finished on an ADA 2019 structure. A clinical case utilizes CPT codes while a dental case utilizes CDT codes. You can cross-code these cases in the event that you're documenting both; however that is a deep, dark hole we won't go down in this article.

The following are a couple of occurrences where you would record clinical protection at your dental practice:

Oral medical procedure

Injury (broken tooth, broken teeth, broken jaw)

Pathology (when the dental specialist performs biopsies expected to check for infections within teeth, gums, and around the mouth)

Obstructive Rest Apnea

Knowing whether to record clinical or dental cases can be extremely confounding, yet here's the uplifting news: you can continuously call and inquire.

This is a typical wellspring of disarray, so if all else fails simply call the clinical and dental insurance agency to affirm which to ship off. On the off chance that you don't settle on a decision and you simply submit dental when it ought to be clinical, you will get a clarification of advantages back that will explain: "Clinical is essential, if it's not too much trouble, submit to clinical and begin the interaction once again."

Clinical protection frequently has an ideal recording breaking point of 3-6 months, rather than the extended opportune documenting limits in numerous dental plans. So you will need to follow clinical cases particularly cautiously to keep away from disavowals because of time limits.

Is dental charging hard to learn?

Dental charging is certainly confounded. To work really hard, it's critical to grasp the entire cycle and make a smooth work process. The obligations included are not abilities that can be mastered in a couple of days.

The cycle begins with gathering the fundamental patient data and entering it accurately. You likewise need to comprehend coding and what connections you should incorporate with your case to be paid. All aspects of the cycle rely upon the past step.

Numerous dental practice proprietors believe that one individual should run the front work area, and deal with all the dental charging. This is normally a recipe for low assortments. Protection charging specifically requires a devoted asset - either an individual, group, or administration zeroed in on gathering installments effectively, particularly from insurance agency.

This is on the grounds that dental charging requires master level information on:

Coordination of advantages rules

Government medical care rules

Step by step instructions to work out a patient's installment obligation

Ascertaining benefits and entering them accurately

Documentation/connections prerequisites for explicit methodology

Step by step instructions to pursue denied claims

Most recent coding refreshes

Posting all installments quickly so your income numbers are correct

Step by step instructions to run reports to show where your charging framework needs consideration

In the event that this feels like a great deal, this is on the grounds that it is! We don't express that to overpower you, just to accentuate the significance of having a specialist set up that can ensure you are gathering all you are owed that can assist the charging with handling run as expected and consistently.

The following are 3 methods for dominating your dental charging:

You may be perusing this reasoning, "Amazing, there's something else to this besides I thought! Where do I start?"

The following are a couple of tips:

1. Keep the dental charging process productive - With regards to your interaction, effectiveness is vital. We referenced a ton of moving parts that should be done precisely, yet additionally as soon as possible. Be precise to cover each charging related task, from booking patients to posting installments. A smooth dental charging process is critical to making a dental practice monetarily sound and compensating everybody fairly. By keeping the expense of gathering installments as low as could be expected, everybody gets the best profit from speculation for their work.

2. Control costs - Investigate how to offload the most costly piece of dental charging: protection claims handling. Tragically, protection charging is in many cases a major consider driving up working expenses. Each neglected case needs follow-up. Sadly, this is difficult to do. Most bustling groups can't stay with up with protection slow down

strategies that save you on hold for quite a long time. Also, there are steady industry changes that are beyond your control:

Government guidelines

State guidelines

CDT coding changes

Insurance contract changes

Patient data

Protection strategies to deny, deferral or minimization installments

You have a decision: Continually screen claims, disavowals, codes and guidelines, strategy updates, and impediments, or have a help keep you on top of this while you regulate.

3. Continue to learn - In light of the fact that medication, insurance contracts, no-pay strategies, and guidelines generally change, dental billers

should constantly be learning. Continually developing your insight and best practices are critical for being a fruitful dental practice. Putting resources into your dental group's schooling and preparing is a decent spot to begin.

Use re-appropriated dental charging to assume command over your dental charging and income

We just tossed a great deal of data at you. What happens next?

Nobody is saying you need to do it all alone. Now that you comprehend how dental charging functions, what the cycle resembles, and how convoluted it can prepare - you're to go after it and enhance it to acquire more cash.

Dental Claim Support is an asset to certainly stand out enough to be noticed dental specialists need on their protection charging. Our master billers can help your group through those confounded COB rules or clinical charging. We can likewise assist your group with smoothing out their cycle to gather more. A decent cycle is the way to high assortments, low expenses, and trust in your income.

Analyzing CDT Code D2940: Do you put defensive reclamations at the crisis arrangement?

A patient presents for a crown planning once the rot is eliminated the discoveries are that the rot stretches out into the mash. The specialist eludes the patient to an endodontist for root trench treatment. The patient is uncertain about whether to continue with the root trench treatment as opposed to having the tooth extricated and an embed put and reestablished with a crown.

Helpful material is set to keep the tooth from breaking further and furthermore to shield the tooth from torment.

We as a whole run into these sorts of patient arrangements where a transitory reclamation is set for different situations. Anyway, how is the arrangement of this supportive material archived and answered to the payer?

Dental Claim Support has fostered our instructive stage; Dental Cases Foundation to address questions, for example, these. Coding and documentation are fundamental for submitting precise protection claims. As a believed dental charging accomplice, we've perceived how instructive devices like Dental Cases Foundation can assist dental groups with keeping awake to date on coding best practices.

In this article, we will look at CDT code D2940 and answer the inquiry: Do you put defensive reclamations at the crisis arrangement? We will likewise cover how to charge for code D2940. This information will assist you with submitting more precise protection claims, prompting more protection income for your dental practice.

What is CDT code D2940?

This kind of reclamation is precisely recorded and answered to the payer utilizing code D2940 which was reexamined a couple of years prior. The past code terminology characterized this code as a soothing filling. The ongoing code language incorporates an overhauled classification and a descriptor.

D2940 defensive reclamation

Direct situation of a helpful material to safeguard tooth or potentially tissue structure. This methodology might be utilized to ease torment, advance recuperating, or forestall further disintegration. Not to be utilized for endodontic access conclusion, or as a base or liner under reclamation.

The classification characterizes D2940 as a defensive rebuilding. The ongoing descriptor further characterizes the expected utilization of the code to give the treating supplier direction for legitimate coding.

It is an immediate reclamation, implying that the rebuilding is put straightforwardly on the tooth, not manufactured external the mouth then, at that point, put on the tooth.

The kind of helpful material isn't indicated. Any kind of helpful material might be utilized when the reason for the arrangement is to safeguard the tooth as well as tissue structure.

Tissue structure insurance could be filling a profound mesial break to hold the tissue back from developing into the broke part of the tooth.

The descriptor then, at that point, proceeds to depict that the reclamation might be utilized to alleviate torment, maybe in a crisis circumstance; advance mending as in the circumstance where the rot might be near the nerve causing uneasiness; or further disintegration of the tooth maybe in the example, the tooth is severely cracked and the rebuilding is put to forestall further breaking of the tooth until authoritative treatment might be performed.

It is likewise vital to take note of the descriptor clarifies what methodology this code isn't suitable for. Code D2940 doesn't record and report reclamation set to close an endodontic access opening. Nor is D2940 to be utilized to report the position of a base or liner.

Per CDT rules, situation of a base or liner is comprehensive to the reclamation and is certainly not a different methodology.

Documentation of defensive reclamation dental methods

For a defensive reclamation, be certain your clinical documentation completely upholds the clinical/dental need of the method. Be explicit in your documentation expressing the state of the tooth requiring the defensive reclamation.

At the end of the day, explicitness in why it is required; the discoveries or determination. What reason does it serve, for example, to alleviate torment in a crisis circumstance? Likewise, incorporate the treatment arranged, as this is definitely not a conclusive treatment, and some other relevant data intended for this patient's treatment.

Is a defensive rebuilding repaid by dental plans?

This is dependably an issue of worry as a dental specialist ought to get compensated for the administrations delivered. While code D2940 isn't a "by report" code, meaning a story isn't needed, it is smart to incorporate an account portraying why the system is fundamental for productive cases settlement (handling).

A fast survey of a couple of dental plans and a couple of PPO handling strategy manuals demonstrate that inclusion changes incredibly. A few plans may possibly pay for D2940 defensive rebuilding when set for help with discomfort in a crisis circumstance. A few plans believe code D2940 to be what is known as a reclaim code.

What is a reclaim code?

At the point when a dental arrangement believes a methodology to be a reclaim, that's what it intends in the event that D2940 is performed and paid by the arrangement, a conclusive reclamation is set inside a predefined time period, then, at that point, the sum paid for the authoritative rebuilding is decreased by the sum paid for D2940. A reclaim code is something you ought to know about for this methodology.

Try not to let coding mistakes hold your dental practice back from being paid

This data is pivotal with regards to running your dental practice. Legitimate coding is straightforwardly connected to not just the moral standard your dental practice is keeping up with yet in addition how much income you are getting.

Your dental practice gets in some cases half of its general income from protection claims, so the income of your dental practice relies upon exact case accommodation.

CDT code D4910: When would it be advisable for me to charge Periodontal Support?

As a dental expert, you knew all about the periodontal support method and CDT code D4910. In any case, applying this code can in any case be confounding.

The descriptor for D4910 gives clear direction with regards to its utilization and what is remembered for the methodology. A few codes contain extensive, itemized descriptors like D4910.

Practice the board programming limits the quantity of characters that can be placed or seen while choosing the right code.

At Dental Claim Support, coding information is profoundly desired in view of what it means for your case accommodation and repayment. We've gone through the beyond couple of years creating Dental Cases Institute to assist dental groups with remaining instructed on points, for example, CDT coding. Accurately coding dental methodology can influence the amount you gather on your protection cases, and it can influence the consistence of your dental practice.

This article resolves 3 of the most often posed inquiries about CDT code D4910. By going through these inquiries, you will have a more profound comprehension of when to charge periodontal upkeep and when to utilize CDT code D4910.

What is CDT code D4910?

We should initially view at the code all in all.

The code states:

D4910 periodontal support

This system is established following periodontal treatment and goes on at, not entirely set in stone by the clinical assessment of the dental specialist, for the existence of the dentition or any embed substitutions. It incorporates evacuation of the bacterial plaque and analytics from supragingival and subgingival locales, site explicit scaling and root planing where demonstrated, and cleaning the teeth. If new or repeating periodontal infection shows up, extra analytic and treatment methodology should be thought of.

When do I utilize CDT code D4910?

The following are 3 every now and again posed inquiries in which the D4910 code could be used:

Question 1: My patient had periodontal support (D4910). She returned multi month after the fact for periodontal scaling and root planing D4342 in one quadrant. Two teeth were dealt with.

Her protection was denied with the explanation being the restricted scaling and root planing is comprehensive to the D4910 methodology performed multi month earlier. Why would that be the situation when the ensuing scaling and root planing was an alternate treatment?

Reply: A survey of the D4910 descriptor states, "It incorporates..., site-explicit scaling and root planing where demonstrated,... ". Most dental plans have a recurrence constraint between any scaling and root planing and periodontal upkeep methods. The most widely recognized recurrence is 90 days.

In the event that the patient's arrangement recurrence limit is 90 days, repayment won't be made. The charge turns into the patient's liability except if a PPO contract restricts charging the patient.

Some PPO contracts incorporate a recurrence restriction. That recurrence PPO arrangement could consider the assistance non-billable to the patient. For instance, some PPOs require 90 days between any scaling and root planing and D4910, very much like dental plans.

On the off chance that the medicines don't meet this necessity, it very well may be a discount for the training. Allude to your PPO handling strategy manuals for clearness on such arrangements.

Question 2: I got a refusal for D4910 because of recurrence. How might I pursue this? My patient is seen for periodontal upkeep 4 times each year. His dental arrangement permits 2 periodontal upkeep methodology and 2 prophylaxis systems each schedule year.

Reply: First, survey the clinical documentation. The documentation ought to show that a prophylaxis was preceded as a feature of the D4910 technique. Per the descriptor, D4910 incorporates "… evacuation of the bacterial plaque and analytics from supragingival and subgingival locales, and cleaning the teeth".

At the point when the documentation upholds a prophylaxis, request the disavowal, and request an elective advantage of a prophylaxis since it was important for the D4910 methodology. An example story is: "On the off chance that D4910 benefits are not accessible, if it's not too much trouble, think about an elective advantage of a grown-up prophylaxis (D1110) as a prophylaxis was preceded as a component of the D4910".

Question 3: A refusal for D4910 was gotten for my patient expressing no set of experiences of periodontal treatment on document. This patient has been getting periodontal upkeep for a considerable length of time.

She just changed positions and has another protection. Her protection expresses that she should have a background marked by scaling and root planing inside the past three years. How could this forswearing be pursued?

Reply: Allure. Demonstrate the date of the last periodontal treatment, for example, scaling and root planing for every quadrant. Another dental arrangement or protection payer will constantly require the last periodontal treatment date since they don't have the set of experiences on record. D4910 is demonstrated following dynamic periodontal treatment, per the descriptor.

Additionally, incorporate authentic complete periodontal diagramming and testing. The account ought to have dates of D4910 and documentation of any site-explicit scaling and root planing proceeded as a feature of the D4910 visits.

The clinical documentation should be well defined for the teeth numbers and locales where scaling and root planing was performed during the D4910 visit. Without explicitness in documentation, chances of winning this sort of allure are not likely.

Prepared to feel more certain while coding?

Documentation is basic in every one of the three models talked about in this article. Particularity in the clinical notes is an unquestionable requirement for all techniques. The absence of subtleties of what was performed and why it was performed is a continuous issue for most dental groups. Consider holding irregular outline reviews in your training collectively.

Utilize the aftereffects of your inner review to learn and work on your documentation. A few payers won't acknowledge a story, just the diagram note for the referred to date of administration. Exhaustiveness in documentation isn't about repayment as much as demonstrating quality patient consideration and clinical need.

Dental Cases Foundation is an asset for dental experts who wish to feel enabled while dealing with their coding and charging. The instructive stage offers courses covering a wide range of subjects, for example, CDT coding, documentation, and charging best practices.

Dental strengths and subspecialties

In many nations that perceive strengths in dentistry, the expert is restricted to rehearse in the forte and can't do the act of general dentistry. Where the specialty is in this way restricted, the overall dental specialist might elude patients and an expert's training is principally on a reference premise. In England and in specific regions in

Canada, experts might lead a general practice. In the US nine strengths are perceived by the American Dental Affiliation: orthodontics and dentofacial muscular health; pediatric dentistry; periodontics; prosthodontics; oral and maxillofacial medical procedure; oral and maxillofacial pathology; endodontics; general wellbeing dentistry; and oral and maxillofacial radiology.

Orthodontics and dentofacial muscular health

Orthodontics takes as its goes for the gold adjustment of malocclusion of the teeth and related dentofacial ambiguities. Orthodontics has been polished since antiquated times, yet strategies for treatment including the utilization of groups and removable machines have been conspicuous just starting from the start of the twentieth 100 years. The US gave driving force to the improvement of orthodontics, which was perceived as a specialty with the development of the American Culture of Orthodontists in 1900.

The interest for this help stretches out from the kid to the full grown-up, albeit human bone answers tooth development best in an individual under 18, and it is for the most part concurred that youngsters benefit more from treatment than do grown-ups. By and large, oral wellbeing and actual appearance are the two most significant explanations behind endeavor a course of orthodontic consideration.

Pediatric dentistry

Pediatric dentistry, similar to pediatrics in medication, is worried about the dental consideration of kids and youths.

A large part of the daily schedule of training is fixated on the control of caries (tooth rot) and includes the utilization of fluoride and dietary and clean guidance. The need to impact tooth positions presents the following most often experienced issue. The rectification of beginning anomalies in tooth arrangement might hinder the need for extensive treatment. Numerous pediatric dental specialists use development affecting strategies to address jaw arrangements. Tolerance and functioning information on youngsters' ways of behaving and youth physical and mental illnesses and infection repercussions are significant capabilities of the pedodontist.

Periodontics

Periodontics is worried about the counteraction, determination, and treatment of illnesses of the periodontal tissues — the tissues that encompass and uphold the teeth. These tissues comprise for the most part of the gums and the jaws and their connected coterminous designs.

The most pervasive periodontal sickness is periodontitis, normally called pyorrhea, a fiery condition typically delivered by nearby aggravations. Periodontitis, if untreated, obliterates the periodontal tissues and is a significant reason for the deficiency of teeth in grown-ups.

The advances of periodontics have been generally in methods of treatment. It is accepted that bacterial plaque, a delicate layer of substances wealthy in microorganisms that sticks to the teeth, is the variable liable for most obliteration of the gums and the tissues encompassing the teeth. Periodontists advocate expulsion of such plaque by a particular routine of controlled cleanliness.

Prosthodontics

Prosthodontics is worried about the rebuilding and support of oral capability, solace, appearance, and wellbeing by the substitution of missing teeth and coterminous tissues with counterfeit substitutes, or prostheses.

Prosthodontists have extraordinary preparation in the development and position of fixed (fixed) and removable apparatuses for the substitution of missing teeth. They likewise develop obturators, prosthetic gadgets intended to deter surrenders in the top of the mouth in instances of congenital fissure. A subspecialty of prosthodontics is maxillofacial prosthetics, which includes with the making of machines, made out of plastic, silicone, or other present day materials, intended to supplant bits of the face and jaws that have been lost as a result of a medical procedure, illness, inborn problems, or mishap.

The legitimate fitting of oral prostheses requires point by point information on the life structures of the head and neck, of the physiology of the neuromuscular framework, and of the study of impediment and jaw developments. It additionally requires expertise in arranging, mouth planning, impression making, enrollment of jaw relations, attempt in methodology, arrangement of the prostheses, and follow-up care.

Oral and maxillofacial medical procedure

Oral medical procedure manages the finding of, and the medical procedure expected by, infections, wounds, and deformities of the human jaws and related structures. The two dental specialists and doctors elude a wide assortment of extraordinary dental issues to the oral specialist. These may incorporate the evacuation of affected and contaminated teeth and the treatment of blisters, cancers, sores, and diseases of the mouth and jaws. Furthermore, there are more mind boggling issues, like jaw and facial wounds, congenital fissure, and congenital fissure.

Oral and maxillofacial pathology

Oral pathology is the investigation of the causes, cycles, and impacts of oral infection, along with the resultant changes of oral design and works.

The oral pathologist gives analyze on which treatment by different experts will depend.

Endodontics

Endodontics manages the treatment of sicknesses of within the tooth, including the mash chamber, the mash channel, and adjacent designs. Root trench treatment and blanching of nonvital teeth are standard medicines delivered by endodontists.

General wellbeing dentistry

General wellbeing dentistry is perceived as a specialty in Canada and the US. The American Dental Affiliation perceives dental general wellbeing as a claim to fame in the event that the holder of the graduate degree continues to a further year of concentrate in preparing and finishes the assessment of the American Leading body of Dental General Wellbeing. Preparing in dental general wellbeing is additionally accessible in the

Assembled Realm. The specialty isn't accentuated similarly in that frame of mind of the world.

Oral and maxillofacial radiology

Oral and maxillofacial radiology manages the utilization of X-beams for conclusion and treatment of infections or issues of the mouth and jaw. It embraces the standard X-beam as well as the panographic X-beam, as well as the utilization of radiation and radioactive materials in therapy of sickness of the mouth and jaws.

Corrective dentistry

The face is the most unmistakable component of an individual. The mouth, which incorporates the lips, cheeks, jaws, teeth, and gums, makes up the lower third of the face. Restorative (or stylish) dentistry might offer significant advantages to the personal satisfaction for those individuals who need it.

Corrective dentistry might be named skeletal or dental. Skeletal changes might be accomplished through oral medical procedure, which can change the place of the jaws. Dental changes might be accomplished by adding to, detracting from, or moving the teeth. The most widely recognized materials to add to teeth to change their appearance are holding, a tooth-hued plastic, or porcelain, a sort of clay. Removing tooth structure is achieved with a drill. If by some stroke of good luck a small measure of the tooth is taken out, it is called chiseling or reshaping, and nothing is in this manner added. On the off chance that a more significant measure of tooth is eliminated, porcelain might be included another position. Moving teeth is achieved with supports, which can be either fixed or removable.

Reconstructive dentistry

Reconstructive dentistry includes any significant remaking of the mouth, ordinarily with porcelain and metal. Reconstructive dentistry might be required by people who have numerous extreme holes, have summed up serious gum sickness, or have been in a mishap. Reconstructive dentistry regularly includes a blend of the relative multitude of dental fortes; patients might require various crowns (covers), gum treatment, root waterway treatment, supports, or oral medical procedure, including dental inserts.

Recreations are intended to initially stop the continuation of dynamic sickness and afterward fix the harm. Profound parts of treatment, like trepidation, are much of the time in question, and a dental specialist should be mindful and have a comprehension of brain research. Significant expected wellsprings of postoperative torment are many times disposed of from the get-go in treatment by performing root waterway treatment when demonstrated. The creation of definite porcelain spans as a rule starts 6 to 12 weeks observing the fulfillment of any important medical procedure. It is basic for patients to comprehend that reproduced teeth require successive cleanings and support.

Embed dentistry

A dental embed is a counterfeit tooth root. It appends counterfeit teeth to the hidden jawbone. Dental inserts might be pictured as screws, and the jawbone might be viewed as a piece of wood. Under this similarity, a screw would be transformed a portion of its length into a piece of wood, and a counterfeit tooth would be stuck to the piece of the screw projecting over the wood. The tooth would be solidly joined to the screw, which thus would be immovably moored in the wood. A solitary dental embed might be utilized for one missing tooth. Four to eight dental inserts might be set in a jaw that is feeling the loss of the relative multitude of teeth.

Dental inserts should be set in a sufficient measure of bone that is liberated from disease. Now and again surgeries are first vital either to wipe out existing contamination or to make more bone for implantation methodology, like bone edge increase or nasal sinus rise. The medical procedure to put the dental inserts themselves is like that of tooth expulsion.

Dental embed reproductions can require 6 to a year to finish, generally in light of the mending time essential between medical procedures. Since bone is living tissue, it needs time to answer well to the biocompatible titanium inserts. The biophysics of the early cell reaction of the hard (bone) and delicate (skin and tendon) tissues to dental implantation is an area of extraordinary exploration and discussion. The advantages of this examination persist to muscular health — for instance, with the substitution of spinal poles and the recuperating of troublesome broken bones, the two of which require screws for guaranteed immobilization.

Embed dentistry has developed into an entirely unsurprising treatment choice for some individuals.

Oral microbial science

Oral microbial science, which is worried about the impacts of the in excess of 600 distinct types of oral microscopic organisms on the teeth, gums, mouth, and different pieces of the body that associate with the mouth through the stomach related framework and the flow, is a significant piece of dental practice. Illness of the teeth and gums is for the most part bacterial in beginning and can significantly affect general wellbeing. For instance, the presence of specific types of microbes in the gums can adversely impact the soundness of the heart and other significant organs.

A lot of examination in dentistry centers on oral microbial science. Immunizations to forestall depressions are being considered, and anti-infection agents are utilized to treat periodontal (gum) illness. Immunizations and anti-toxins work by smothering or killing explicit types of microbes that have been distinguished as causative specialists of illness.

Geriatric dentistry

Geriatric dentistry is worried about the oral wellbeing of older people, who normally have huge clinical issues and are taking various prescriptions. Furthermore, they might have mental and financial issues that require complex dental administration. A fundamental reason of geriatric dentistry is that old individuals frequently experience side effects of dental rot and gingival (gum) messes that vary from side effects experienced by more youthful individuals. Dental treatment for the old is accordingly equipped to any physical and mental impediments they might have.

Unfortunate oral wellbeing in the old can prompt loss of hunger, ailing health, metabolic issues, and even, in instances of facial deformation, the beginning of misery. Periodontal infection has been connected to coronary illness, stroke, diabetes, osteoporosis, and different sicknesses. With the quantity of old people of old age (85 years or more seasoned) with mental problems, for example, Alzheimer sickness arriving at pandemic extents, dental administration of impacted people has turned into a significant test in clinical dental practice. The old frequently take numerous drugs, which have unfavorable secondary effects like dry mouth, a significant reason for dental rot. The impacts of maturing bring about changes in lip pose, biting proficiency, and capacity to swallow and taste and in an expansion in sicknesses of the hard and delicate tissues of the mouth.

Albeit most of the older hold their normal teeth, dental rot, periodontal sickness, and loss of teeth in people beyond 65 years old have arrived at critical extents. This accumulation of oral issues requests schooling, research, and high level clinical preparation in geriatric dentistry.

Different disciplines

There are a few different disciplines in dentistry that, albeit false claims to fame or subspecialties, are by and by the chief main subject area of different dental specialists, who give all or a significant piece of their training to these fields. Among them are oral medication and criminological dentistry.

Oral medication, or stomatology, treats the range of illnesses that influence both the skin and the oral mucous films. A portion of these sicknesses, for example, pemphigus vulgaris, can foster their most memorable signs in the mouth and can life-undermine. Oral malignant growth likewise has a high death rate, mostly in light of the fact that it fills in such closeness to such countless essential designs and promptly includes them. With all such illnesses of the oral pit, evacuation of a part of the sore for assessment under the magnifying instrument (biopsy) by an oral pathologist is a fundamental technique, and numerous other research center strategies are frequently likewise expected for the conclusion of oral mucosal sicknesses.

Criminological dentistry is the review and practice of parts of dentistry that are applicable to lawful issues. It is a specialty polished by not many and isn't generally essential for dental schooling. Criminological dentistry is, in any case, of significant lawful significance because of multiple factors, one of the most significant of which is the way that the teeth are the designs of the body generally impervious to fire or festering. Also, the game plan of the teeth or any reclamation in them is essentially or totally special to some random individual and, on the off chance that dental records can be found, may empower distinguishing proof with sureness like that given by fingerprinting. For instance, the recognizable proof of human remaining parts after airplane mishaps can frequently be made exclusively by this implies. Minor anomalies of the teeth can likewise be repeated in indentations, which empower a suspect to be distinguished on the off chance that the person in question has chomped someone else.

Dental instruction

Predental programs

In a larger part of nations on the planet, undergrad preparing in dentistry is accessible. Many require predental preparing before acknowledgment into a school of dentistry. The predental preparing is notwithstanding essential and optional training, which typically takes from 10 to 12 years. The expected number of years in predental schooling changes from one to seven (various European nations expect from five to seven years of clinical training prior to entering dentistry). Predental course preparing generally incorporates such examinations as science, science, physical science, and math. Certain resources of dentistry in Canada and the US require a four year certification in expressions or science as an essential for entrance into dental personnel.

Dental school and preparing

After predental courses, preparing comprises of four years in a staff of dentistry to qualify as a specialist of dental medical procedure (D.D.S.) or specialist of dental medication (D.M.D.), the two degrees being same. The program of studies during the four-year course incorporates the accompanying natural sciences: human life systems, organic chemistry, bacteriology, histology, pathology, pharmacology, microbial science, and physiology, whereupon the succeeding investigations of the hypothesis and procedures of dental practice are based. Studies expected regarding dental practice incorporate supportive dentistry, prosthetics, orthodontics, medical procedure, preventive dentistry, medication, dental general wellbeing, pedodontics, periodontics, radiology, clinical practice, and sedation.

Auxiliary dental fields

Dental hygienists

The dental hygienist is a figure in the mission to lessen periodontal illness and to work on actual prosperity by advancing better consideration of the mouth.

The avoidance of oral sickness through schooling and therapy is the central capability of hygienists. The particular obligations and administrations that they are permitted to perform rely upon the local laws of the authorizing bodies, the prerequisites of the dental workplaces, in which they are utilized, or the points and targets of the general wellbeing programs in which they are locked in. Hygienists for the most part work under the compelling oversight of a certified dental specialist. At times, hygienists are allowed to work without oversight.

Hygienists utilized in dental workplaces eliminate stores and stains from the patient's teeth; apply fluorides, and notice and record states of rot and illness for the dental specialist's data. Further obligations might incorporate the taking of X-beam photos of parts of the mouth, which the hygienist creates and mounts. One more capability of the hygienist is to advance dental wellbeing by prompting on diet and nourishment and empowering oral cleanliness.

Hygienists utilized by instructive specialists help school dental specialists by performing such obligations as analyzing youngsters' teeth. They may likewise visit homerooms to make sense of the significance of oral cleanliness and to give guidance in the legitimate consideration of the teeth and gums. In emergency clinics they perform for the most part similar obligations concerning private experts.

Dental medical attendants and dental assistants

In New Zealand, helpers known as dental medical attendants (or dental specialists) have been doing a dental consideration program for youngsters for various years. Customarily, a dental medical attendant gets insignificant management however is prepared to give a dental consideration program to kids and youths as long as 18 years old. Before, a degree in dental treatment required two years of specific preparation. Today a college level Lone ranger of Oral Wellbeing degree has supplanted programs in dental treatment in New Zealand. To get an unhitched male's in oral wellbeing, understudies are prepared in both dental treatment and dental cleanliness.

Dental collaborators

Most of dental specialists in confidential practice utilize at least one dental collaborator to offer such types of assistance as the gathering of patients, the keeping of records and records, help for the dental specialist while the person in question is treating patients, general upkeep of the workplace, creating of dental X-beams, and sanitization of instruments.

Dental innovation

Dental experts, additionally called dental mechanics, make counterfeit crowns, scaffolds, false teeth, and other dental apparatuses as per dental specialists' determinations. Work orders, joined by models or impressions of patients' mouths; express the specific prerequisites for every specific work. In huge research centers the different phases of production are frequently partitioned, and the experts utilized may practice. Now and then to some extent talented people are employed to work in restricted parts of creation on a sequential construction system premise.

Associations

In the US, each state has its own dental society, which is partitioned into neighborhood social orders. Enrollment in the nearby society consequently presents participation in the state society and the American Dental Affiliation. What's more, the Public Dental Affiliation exists to address ethnic minorities in dentistry in the US. The Public Dental Affiliation was shaped in 1932 by African American dental specialists, who were encountering racial separation and were kept from becoming individuals from coordinated dental social orders. Today the American Dental Affiliation will permit no type of racial inclination to forestall enrollment. Dental specialists with comparable interests have framed their own associations, like the American Relationship of Ladies Dental specialists, the Public Relationship of Seventh Day Adventist Dental specialists, the American Institute of the Historical backdrop of Dentistry, and numerous others. Also, every specialty has its own association.

Relationship of dental specialists, dental diaries, and dental schools exist in pretty much every nation of the world. The Fédération Dentaire Internationale (Worldwide Dental Alliance) was established in 1900 and has met yearly besides in the midst of war. It has supported worldwide dental congresses that are intended to meet at regular intervals. Other global associations incorporate the Affiliation Internationale pour la Recherche Dentaire (Worldwide Relationship for Dental Exploration) and the Affiliation pour les Recherches sur les Paradentopathies (Relationship for Examination into Periodontal Illnesses), which was coordinated in 1932. The Global Dental Diary, distributed by the Fédération Dentaire Internationale, was established in 1950.

Inside the overall structure of the World Wellbeing Association, the dental wellbeing program has advanced consistently all along. A proposition for a joint survey of stomatology and dental cleanliness as a team with the Fédération Dentaire Internationale was made at the main World Wellbeing Get together in 1948.

Certain associations, including the World Wellbeing Association and the Fédération Dentaire Internationale, and nations, for example, New Zealand and the US offer help to many emerging nations in the arrangement of wellbeing instructive and dental consideration administrations. For instance, New Zealand has long provided non-industrial nations with the advantage of its involvement with the utilization of dental helpers, or what are generally known as school dental medical caretakers. Direct help is given in the advancement of other general wellbeing dental administrations to nations like Sri Lanka, Malaysia, Singapore, Brunei, Thailand, Indonesia, and Papua New Guinea. Dental specialists from these nations have had the valuable chance to concentrate on the New Zealand framework, and various school dental medical attendants have accepted their preparation there, empowering them to aid the foundation of preparing offices in their nations of origin.

Blood donation center, association that gathers stores, processes, and bonds blood. During The Second Great War it was shown the way that put away blood could securely be utilized, considering the advancement of the principal blood donation center in 1932. Before the primary blood donation centers came into activity, a doctor decided the blood classifications of the patient's family members and companions until the legitimate kind was found, played out the crossmatch, drained the benefactor, and gave the bonding to the patient. During the 1940s the disclosure of many blood classifications and of a few cross matching methods prompted the fast improvement of blood banking as a particular field and to a progressive shift of liability regarding the specialized parts of bonding from rehearsing doctors to experts and clinical pathologists. The reasonableness of putting away new endlessly blood parts for future necessities made conceivable such advancements as counterfeit kidneys, heart-lung siphons for open-heart medical procedure, and trade bondings for babies with erythroblastosis fetalis.

Entire blood is given and put away in units of around 450 ml (somewhat short of what one 16 ounces). Entire blood can be put away just temporarily, yet different parts (e.g., red platelets and plasma) can be frozen and put away for a year or longer. Hence, most blood gifts are isolated and put away as parts by the blood donation center.

These parts incorporate platelets to control dying; concentrated red platelets to address paleness; and plasma divisions, for example, fibrinogen to help thickening, resistant globulins to forestall and treat various irresistible sicknesses, and serum egg whites to expand the blood volume in instances of shock. In this way, serving the fluctuating requirements of at least five patients with a solitary blood donation is conceivable.

Notwithstanding such substitution programs, many blood donation centers deal with ceaseless issues in acquiring adequate gifts. The constant lack of contributors has been mitigated to some degree by the improvement of apheresis, a procedure by which just an ideal blood part is taken from the giver's blood, with the leftover liquid and platelets promptly bonded once more into the benefactor. This strategy permits the assortment of a lot of a specific part, like plasma or platelets, from a solitary contributor.

Spa, spring or resort with warm or mineral water utilized for drinking and washing. The name was taken from a town close to Liège, Belg., to which people went for the presumed corrective properties of its mineral springs.

The act of "taking the waters" for restorative purposes arrived at its prime in the nineteenth hundred years, however springs have been viewed as spots of mending at ordinarily and in all areas of the planet. The establishing of Shower in Britain is ascribed in legend to Bladud, child of Lud Hudibras and father of Lord Lear, who in 863 BC was restored of sickness by drenching in the steaming bogs. Roman settlers fostered an impressive spa there and furthermore at Buxton, Derbyshire. After the flight of the Romans the showers appear to have been for quite some time dismissed, however many houses of worship were based on destinations of antiquated spots of mending all through Europe, and fixes were ascribed to drenching in textual styles took care of by the springs underneath the safe-haven. In the mid eighteenth century a few Roman showers were remade, some new "watering places" were laid out, and spas became popular mainstream communities of resort for the privileged society's at the most convenient seasons. For the evil and weak numerous spas gave all year therapy focuses under changing levels of clinical oversight.

Spa treatment depends on both the drinking of and the washing in specific waters containing properties accepted to be of restorative worth. Mineral springs typically contain observable amounts of salts in arrangement — including carbonate and sulfate of lime, normal salt, iron, and sulfur. Magnesia and many minor elements, strikingly lithium, likewise comprise therapeutic waters. Notwithstanding strong constituents, gas is available in many waters in significant amounts. There is a little oxygen and a fair setup of nitrogen in some of them. The amount of hydrosulfuric corrosive, even areas of strength for in waters, is little; however the volume of carbonic corrosive present is many times enormous, giving perceptible foam. Warm springs are gotten from two sources: fleeting waters that ascent from extensive profundities along crevices of entrance; and volcanic waters, which arrive at the surface as either fountains or natural aquifers. Most warm water contains mineral substance in arrangement.

The spas of Europe and the US with the best ubiquity were those with warm springs. Washing in warm water has an undoubted helpful impact as a guide to unwinding, albeit the skin doesn't retain any of the salts or gases. Sulfurated waters like those at Aachen, Ger., Baden, Austria, and White Sulfur Springs, W.Va., are utilized for some skin conditions. Drinking mineral waters may, at any rate, give a general cleaning out of the stomach related framework, and the basic waters of Vichy,

Fr., Ischia, Italy, and Mariánské Lázně, Czech Republic, may go about as laxative specialists. The profoundly carbonated salt springs at Saratoga Springs, N.Y., and at Wiesbaden and Baden, Ger., have for some time been utilized for rheumatic and neuralgic circumstances. Drinking mineral water, carbonated or not, has become so well known that an impressive business of restraining and trading has developed on the two sides of the Atlantic; it has a viable significance in helping processing that is a lot more prominent than one would anticipate from its little mineral substance.

It is reasonable, nonetheless, that the vast majority of the restorative impacts of spa treatment result from the ecological elements of the area and offices of the spa. The lovely town of Shower has the main warm springs in Britain, which typically yields in excess of 500,000 gallons day to day at a temperature of 120° F (49° C). The waters are plastered restoratively and utilized for hydrotherapy medicines, and the Georgian Siphon Room, with its wellspring, has for quite some time been a meeting for guests who are "taking the waters." Numerous European spas are situated in forested snowcapped settings like Sankt Moritz, Switz., Évian-les-Bains, Fr., Badgastein, Austria, and Bormio, Italy. Japan has a few thousand underground aquifers, a large number of which have been changed over into spas or public showers.

A person who goes to a spa for the most part tracks down an alternate environment, diet, and way of living than he is utilized to. In a new and most likely lively society, an individual is looser and may take more practice in the outside. For some people the treatment of the waters is optional to the organization where they are taken, and it has for quite some time been so at spas. After the American Nationwide conflict a spa at French Lick, Ind., delighted in tremendous fame as a gathering spot to organize relationships. Saratoga Springs declined as a spa in the mid twentieth century yet draws in a great many guests to its racecourse every year. For the sick and recuperating numerous spas offer clinical treatment, and for all people the spa has been and keeps on being in various ways a position of mending.

Muscular health, likewise called muscular medical procedure, clinical specialty worried about the protection and reclamation of capability of the skeletal framework and its related designs, i.e., spinal and different bones, joints, and muscles.

The term muscular health was presented in 1741 by French doctor Nicolas Andry de Bois-Respect in his work L'Orthopédie, which highlighted an etching of a warped tree supported with a post and a rope that later turned into an image of the field.

The act of muscular health was spearheaded in the following a long time by Jean André Venel, who laid out an organization in Switzerland for the treatment of disabled kids' skeletal deformations. Boundlessly expanded information on strong capabilities and of the development and improvement of bone was acquired in the nineteenth hundred years. Huge advances as of now were the new activity of tenotomy (the cutting of ligaments, which made revising distortions more straightforward), the careful rectification of clubfoot, the development of the Thomas brace (which offered better help for cracks of long bones in the appendages), and the presentation of fast setting mortar of Paris for use in muscular gauzes. The endeavors of Sir Robert Jones and the gigantic losses from The Second Great War prompted the establishing of numerous muscular instructional hubs in the mid twentieth 100 years.

Present day muscular health has reached out past the treatment of cracks, broken bones, stressed muscles, torn tendons and ligaments, and other horrendous wounds to manage many obtained and inborn skeletal deformations and with the impacts of degenerative illnesses like osteoarthritis. A specialty that initially relied upon the utilization of weighty supports and supports, muscular health presently uses bone unions and fake plastic joints for the hip and different bones harmed by infection, as well as counterfeit appendages, unique footwear, and supports to return versatility to crippled patients. Muscular health utilizes the methods of actual medication and restoration and word related treatment notwithstanding those of customary medication and medical procedure.

Obstetrics and gynecology, clinical/careful specialty worried about the consideration of ladies from pregnancy until after conveyance and with the conclusion and treatment of issues of the female regenerative parcel.

The clinical consideration of pregnant ladies (obstetrics) and of female genital sicknesses (gynecology) created along various verifiable ways. Obstetrics had for quite a while been the region of female birthing specialists (see maternity care), however in the seventeenth 100 years, European doctors started to go to on ordinary conveyances of imperial and distinguished families; from that start, the training developed and spread to the working classes. The development of the forceps utilized in conveyance, the presentation of sedation, and Ignaz Semmelweis' disclosure of the reason for puerperal ("childbed") fever and his presentation of germ-free techniques in the conveyance room were all significant advances in obstetrical practice. Asepsis thus made cesarean segment, in which the baby is conveyed through a cut in the mother's uterus and stomach wall, a doable careful option in contrast to regular labor. By the mid nineteenth hundred years, obstetrics had become laid out as a perceived clinical discipline in Europe and the US.

In the twentieth hundred years, obstetrics grew predominantly in the space of ripeness control and the advancement of sound births. The pre-birth care and guidance of pregnant moms to lessen birth deformities and issue conveyances was presented around 1900 and was from that point quickly embraced all through the world. Starting with the improvement of hormonal preventative pills during the 1950s, obstetrician-gynecologists have likewise become progressively answerable for controlling ladies' fruitfulness and fertility. With the improvement of amniocentesis, ultrasound, and different strategies for the pre-birth conclusion of birth surrenders, obstetrician-gynecologists have had the option to cut short inadequate embryos and undesirable pregnancies.

Simultaneously, new techniques for misleadingly embedding prepared undeveloped organisms inside the uterus have empowered obstetrician-gynecologists to assist already fruitless couples with having kids.

The obstetrician's principal undertakings are to analyze and bring a lady through pregnancy, convey her kid, and give the new mother sufficient post pregnancy care. The main careful activity performed by obstetricians is cesarean area. Episiotomy, a surgery in which a cut is utilized to broaden the vaginal opening to work with labor, is likewise normal.

Gynecology as a part of medication traces all the way back to Greco-Roman human progress, while possibly not prior. The reestablishment of interest in sicknesses of ladies is displayed in the tremendous reference book of gynecology gave in 1566 by Caspar Wolf of Zürich. In the early and mid-nineteenth 100 years, doctors became ready to play out a restricted assortment of careful procedure on the ovaries and uterus effectively. The American specialist James Marion Sims and different trailblazers of usable gynecology likewise needed to battle the fierce bias of the general population against any openness or assessment of the female sexual organs. The two extraordinary advances that at last conquered such resistance and made gynecologic medical procedure by and large accessible were the utilization of sedation and germicide strategies. The different specialty of gynecology had become genuinely deeply grounded by 1880; its association with the specialty of obstetrics, emerging from a cross-over of regular worries, started late in the 100 years and has proceeded to the current day.

Gynecologists make routine assessments of cervical and vaginal emissions to recognize malignant growth of the uterus and cervix. They perform two principal kinds of careful activities:

fixing any huge wounds caused to the vagina, uterus, and bladder throughout labor; and eliminating sores and harmless or dangerous growths from the uterus, cervix, and ovaries. The cutting edge practice of gynecology requires expertise in pelvic medical procedure, information on female urologic conditions, in light of the fact that the side effects of sicknesses of the urinary parcel and the genital plot are frequently comparative, and expertise in managing the minor mental issues that frequently emerge among gynecologic patients.

Comprehensive medication, a convention of preventive and helpful medication that underlines the need of taking a gander at the entire individual — his body, psyche, feelings, and climate — instead of at a confined capability or organ and which advances the utilization of an extensive variety of wellbeing practices and treatments. It has particularly come to pressure liability regarding "self-recuperating," or "taking care of oneself," by noticing the customary realistic basics of activity, stimulating eating routine, sufficient rest, great air, balance in private propensities, etc.

The term comprehensive medication turned out to be particularly popular in the late twentieth hundred years (the Worldwide Relationship of All-encompassing Wellbeing Specialists was established in 1970, accepting at least for a moment that its ongoing all-encompassing name in 1981). In its fundamental way of thinking, in underscoring the arrangement of entire consideration to an individual or patient, all-encompassing medication isn't new, being indistinguishable from any customary medical care of good quality. Comprehensive medication in outrageous occasions, be that as it may, has would in general compare the legitimacy of a large number of schools or ways to deal with medical services, not every one of them viable and some of them serious, some logical and some informal. Despite the fact that standard Western clinical practices are not overlooked, they are viewed as just a single piece of the accessible treatments and in no way, shape or form the main compelling ones. Congresses and meetings on comprehensive wellbeing have in this manner drawn delegates of clinical schools and establishments as well as promoters of such broadly differing ideas as needle therapy, elective labor, soothsaying, biofeedback, chiropractic, confidence recuperating, graphology, homeopathy, macrobiotics, megavitamin treatment, naturopathy, numerology, nourishment, osteopathy, psychocalisthenics, psychotherapy, self-back rub, shiatsu (or pressure point massage), contact experience, and yoga.

Pathology, clinical specialty worried about the deciding reasons for illness and the primary and useful changes happening in strange circumstances. Early endeavors to concentrate on pathology were much of the time obstructed by strict restrictions against dissections, yet these steadily loose during the late Medieval times, permitting post-mortems to decide the reason for death, the reason for pathology. The resultant collecting physical data finished in the distribution of the primary methodical course book of grim life structures by the Italian Giovanni Battista Morgagni in 1761, which found sicknesses inside individual organs interestingly. The connection between's clinical side effects and obsessive changes was not made until the main portion of the nineteenth 100 years.

The current humoral speculations of pathology were supplanted by a more logical cell hypothesis; Rudolf Virchow in 1858 contended that the idea of sickness could be perceived through the tiny examination of impacted cells. The bacteriologic hypothesis of sickness grew late in the nineteenth 100 years by Louis Pasteur and Robert Koch gave the last hint to understanding numerous illness processes.

Pathology as a different specialty was genuinely deeply grounded toward the nineteenth century's end. The pathologist does a lot of his work in the research center and reports to and talks with the clinical doctor who straightforwardly takes care of the patient. The kinds of lab examples inspected by the pathologist incorporate precisely eliminated body parts, blood and other body liquids, pee, excrement, exudates, and so on. Pathology practice likewise incorporates the reproduction of the last section of the genuine life of a departed individual through the methodology of dissection, which gives significant and generally hopeless data concerning infection processes. The information expected for the legitimate general act of pathology is too perfect to be in any way achievable by single people, so any place conditions license it, subspecialist's team up.

Among the research center subspecialties in which pathologists work are neuropathology, pediatric pathology, general careful pathology, dermatopathology, and measurable pathology.

Microbial societies for the ID of irresistible illness, less difficult admittance to interior organs for biopsy using glass fiber-optic instruments, better meaning of subcellular structures with the electron magnifying lens, and a wide exhibit of synthetic stains have significantly extended the data accessible to the pathologist in deciding the reasons for sickness. Formal clinical schooling with the fulfillment of a M.D. degree or its identical is expected preceding admission to pathology postgraduate projects in numerous Western nations. The program expected for board confirmation as a pathologist generally sums to five years of postgraduate review and preparing.

Workmanship treatment, the utilization of innovative flows for of supporting one's prosperity.

Workmanship treatments permit people to put themselves out there through inventive means. Frequently the most common way of making craftsmanship is the center of the course of craftsmanship treatment: through the work, people can encounter themselves as engaged, esteemed, ready to accomplish, and ready to manage an errand. Workmanship can explain profound sentiments and can carry oblivious issues to the front. Bunch workmanship treatment approaches can likewise encourage social communication.

Most craftsmanship rehearses — including dance, music, theater, drawing, photography, mold, and experimental writing — have particular workmanship treatment approaches related with them. One huge contrast between "standard" workmanship practices and craftsmanship treatment is the situation with the end result: ideas like authority, control, and business esteem are either not significant or substantially less significant than self-articulation. Additionally, public utilization isn't really a point of craftsmanship treatment. Public presentation can restoratively affect people, especially individuals who have viewed themselves as being cheapened or invalid, yet the cycles and results of workmanship treatment are additionally private and frequently remain so.

Against both standard practice and craftsmanship treatment approaches stands local area or participatory workmanship practice. There preparing is likewise immaterial, and process frequently is worried about item as a worth by its own doing. Unique in relation to craftsmanship treatment, however, local area and participatory practices frequently pressure the local area as the focal point of the work rehearses. Accomplishing something together and tracking down approaches to communicating a common vision become significant ideas in that workmanship practice, and public showcase is many times seen as powerful in local area changes.

Craftsmanship treatment approaches can be valuable in permitting individuals to manage social marks of shame or individual issues related with physical or mental debilitation. Craftsmanship treatment likewise will in general be the primary spot where regulated individuals experience the option expressive method for workmanship, empowering them to find new points of view on their background.

Word related medication, previously called modern medication, the part of medication worried about the support of wellbeing and the counteraction and treatment of sicknesses and unintentional wounds in working populaces in the working environment. By and large, word related medication was restricted to the treatment of wounds and illnesses happening to creation laborers while at work. Throughout the long term, this changed, with workers at plants, production lines, and workplaces becoming qualified for clinical benefits. School or school wellbeing projects may be considered as expansions of word related medication.

Sicknesses straightforwardly connected with occupations were perceived by early Egyptian and Roman doctors. Present day word related medication might be said to have begun with Bernardino Ramazzini, an Italian doctor of the seventeenth century who unequivocally prompted that the doctor who wished to find out about the causation of a patient's grievance ought to ask into the occupations of the patient. With the Modern Upset the quantity of people presented to expected risks at work expanded quickly. Horrible wounds became successive, and illnesses because of breathed in cleans and toxic gases and fumes were perceived, frequently by nonmedical people.

At first, word related clinical projects were coordinated toward the treatment of wounds or illnesses that came about because of or during work. It was soon evident that avoidance was more conservative than treatment. Defensive gadgets were created and put around moving pieces of apparatus. Control programs were created by specialists to eliminate destructive tidies and fumes by legitimate ventilation of workspaces or by replacement of less poisonous materials. At the point when the designers had zero control over the climate, the cycle was contained to forestall or if nothing else limit the openness of laborers. If all else fails, defensive gadgets, for example, covers and extraordinary apparel were worn by the specialists.

With the advancement of preventive controls, how much word related infection diminished. The advancement of new cycles and new materials, be that as it may, delivered new dangers at an always expanding rate, and steady watchfulness was essential. For instance, the acknowledgment that a pneumonic infection can result from openness to beryllium showed the requirement for a proceeded with consciousness of possibly harmful materials. It likewise showed that a material once remembered to be nontoxic may really be harmful; this shift might be brought about by an adjustment of the physical or synthetic qualities of the material, a modification in the technique by which the material is utilized, an adjustment of how much openness of people to the material, and conceivable synergism with different materials.

The worry with illnesses because of occupation prompted worry with the overall strength of laborers, not just in view of an interest in their government assistance yet in addition since it was great business. A decent word related clinical program further developed work the executives relations and diminished truancy; work turnover diminished and efficiency expanded. In many cases, the reserve funds delivered by the decrease in charges paid for laborers' pay protection paid for the word related clinical program. Contingent upon the nation and the occupation, the kinds of wellbeing programs shift significantly; huge organizations, for instance, will generally offer wide inclusion, while little plants might have restricted clinical projects. The complete projects, as well as giving treatment of infections and wounds, could incorporate pre-work assessments and intermittent assessments during business.

All through the world there is deficient information and announcing of word related infection, and the information are suspect. Distributed figures for word related sicknesses, for example, are more modest than for wounds since event of occupation related disease is less breathtaking than, for instance, a blast of a mine causing various passings. It might require various long stretches of perception and research to find that some specific residue, substance, or kind of actual energy is unsafe.

Also, doctors might experience issues in concluding that an ailment is owing to the gig. Numerous word related infections emulate disorder from different causes, and little is known about the evil impacts and indications of proceeded with little openings to poisonous synthetic substances. Another trouble emerges from the way that in spite of the fact that work related illness might be thought, specialists frequently need tests to recognize such sickness as unambiguous. Thus, against each analyzed instance of word related sickness, there might be numerous nascent or unnoticed cases from similar causes. Presentation of materials of obscure poisonousness, as well as changes in modern tasks, may make unnoticed issues in forestalling destructive impacts until after specialists have been impacted.

Horace Wells, (conceived January 21, 1815, Hartford, Vermont, U.S. — passed on January 24, 1848, New York, New York), American dental specialist, a trailblazer in the utilization of careful sedation.

While rehearsing in Hartford, Connecticut, in 1844, Wells noticed the torment killing properties of nitrous oxide ("snickering gas") during a giggling gas street show and from that point involved it in performing easy dental tasks. He was permitted to exhibit the strategy at the Massachusetts General Emergency clinic in January 1845, yet when the patient moaned, driving spectators to presume that the patient felt aggravation, Wells was presented to mock.

After William Morton, a dental specialist and Wells' previous accomplice, effectively exhibited ether sedation in October 1846, Wells started broad self-trial and error with nitrous oxide, ether, chloroform, and different synthetic compounds to discover their relative sedative properties. His character fundamentally changed by successive inward breath of substance fumes, he was imprisoned in New York City for tossing corrosive at bystanders. There, in a prison cell, he ended his own life while the Paris Clinical Society was freely acclaiming him the pioneer of sedative gases.

Protection and Medication

People, associations and legislatures esteem and safeguard clinical protection (Francis and Francis 2017; Beauchamp and Childress 2008; Humber and Almeder 2001; Englehardt 2000b). When in doubt, they endeavor to (1) limit and secure what they consider to be delicate clinical data and biospecimens, (2) regard therapeutically related choices by people and families and (3) honor local area and lawful assumptions for protection

(Francis 2017; Winslade 2014). For over fifty years, scholars and bioethicists have taken a strong fascination with security issues. They have added to a growing writing, some with commonsense applications, comprising of different points of view on how security ideas and values are ensnared in persistent consideration and biomedical examination (Official Commission 2012).

The extent of this passage is "protection" in the few shifted and famous purposes of the term utilized in medication and wellbeing research, including the disputable purposes bantered by rationalists. Most contemporary conversations of protection and medication concern the enlightening security of patients and exploration subjects, treated in Area 1, underneath. Clinical record classification is an incessant concentration. This accentuation is neither astonishing nor unseemly given the issues, needs and distractions of the computerized age. Not to be neglected, and canvassed here in Segments 2 and 5, scholarly conversation has stretched out past educational protection, drawing in the security ramifications of noticing, contacting and deciding for oneself in clinical practice. These types of protection are in some cases alluded to as physical and decisional security. Associational and exclusive ideas of security found in wellbeing related dicussions and perceived by certain thinkers are additionally momentarily treated in beneath in Segments 3 and 4.

This passage mainly manages the expert work of doctors, attendants and other prepared and authorized clinical guardians, alongside medical clinics, insurance agency and specialists. Protection comparable to health and prosperity are past the extent of this passage, but to the impressive degree that it prompts experiences with clinical experts and associations. Wellbeing experiences with profound, wellness or non-clinical excellence experts are not examined. At last, while the security of patients and biomedical examination subjects is the focal point of this passage, philosophical inquiries concerning wellbeing experts' own protection related interests embroiled in clinical practice are perceived.

1. Enlightening Protection

This segment will feature philosophical issues connecting with instructive security and medication. In clinical settings, the "security" at issue is frequently "secrecy" (DeCew 2000). Medical services experts recognize moral obligations to keep clinical data hidden (APA 2017; AAMFT 2015). Doctors, medical attendants, emergency clinics, drug specialists, and safety net providers are legally necessary and expert codes to rehearse classification. Since the 1990s, in arrangement conversations of wellbeing strategy and change, worries about secrecy have frequently been conspicuous (Sharpe 2005; Schwartz 1995). Secrecy rehearses stay notable in clinical settings, even as individuals from the overall population show more loosened up perspectives about willfully sharing wellbeing and clinical data.

A couple of fundamental focuses about enlightening security and medication bear accentuation toward the beginning — one about open perspectives, a second about proficient obligation, a third about regulation and strategy, and a fourth about the meaning of inconsistencies and enormous information examination to significant clinical protection.

To start with, while data sharing has developed more normal in late many years — due, entomb alia, to online entertainment, enormous information, accuracy medication, and expanded irresistible illness, new medication showcasing and other wellbeing reconnaissance — people generally remain quiet about some wellbeing concerns, whether out of private inclination, moral save, behavior, dread or disgrace (Allen 2016; Rosenberg 2000; Buss 1980; Westin 1967). At the point when they share what they consider touchy wellbeing worries with others, most people utilize socially suitable carefulness and save (Nissenbaum 2009; Goffman 1959, 1963). In light of such security rehearses, families, companions, managers, representatives, colleagues, specialists, scientists and legislatures may not gain all the clinical data they need, when they need it (Currie 2005; Etzioni 2000). Simultaneously, people who need clinical security might feel they need significant command over what befalls their own data. The ascent of web-based entertainment, PDAs, wearable wellbeing observing gadgets, individual ownership of electronic duplicates of clinical records, buyer DNA testing and accuracy medication address different open doors for expected and accidental divulgences of wellbeing related pictures and data. The useful capacity of people to control and safeguard their wellbeing protection is halfway an element of powerful information security, their insight into contemporary clinical information the executives practices and social-financial honors (Extensions 2017; Marx 2007). Kids, alongside grown-ups in dynamic military assistance, made a decision about intellectually clumsy, subject to government qualification programs or imprisoned, need significant command over their clinical security (Annas et al. 2013). With regards to health related crises, contaminations sicknesses and plagues, able grown-up regular folks not in care might be denied the decision to keep their clinical data hidden.

Second, numerous clinical experts, clinics, guarantors and different substances with admittance to wellbeing data respect keeping up with the secrecy of clinical correspondences and the security of clinical data as foremost expert obligations (Daly et al., 2015; Official

Commission 2016). This reasonableness reaches out to social work, emotional wellness and drug store records. Additionally, clinical medical services suppliers and bio-clinical scientists by and large look to oblige patients' sensible assumptions for protection and are expected to do as such by state and public regulations (Allen 2011; Official Commission 2009). All things considered, empowering patients to embrace sharing wellbeing data to further develop research, clinical practices and their own consideration is a new pattern (Juengst et al. 2016).

Third, social orders force significant protection and confidential decision related legitimate commitments on their individuals (Waldman 2018; Allen 2016; Westin 1967). Lawful commitments of protection and secrecy tie people and furthermore tie medical care suppliers, guarantors, wellbeing information processors, wellbeing analysts, general wellbeing authorities and government (Mello at al. 2016; DHHS 2015; GAO 2001). In this way in various general sets of laws, uncovering a confidential clinical truth or breaking clinical classification can bring about common obligation (Allen and Rotenberg 2016; Solove 2004, 2008). The law forces commitments to regard educational protection (e.g., classification, obscurity, mystery and information security); actual protection (e.g., unobtrusiveness and substantial honesty); associational security (e.g., private sharing of death, ailment and recuperation); restrictive security (e.g., self-possession and command over private identifiers, hereditary information, and biospecimens); and decisional protection (e.g., independence and decision in clinical navigation) (Allen 2016). However security isn't everything in that frame of mind of the law, nor is it an adequate or outright moral great (Allen 2003). With regards to crises and general wellbeing emergencies, for example, the Coronavirus worldwide pandemic, side effect checking, exposures, reconnaissance and contact following that decrease security might be supported and lawfully allowed or commanded. The craving of wellbeing authorities and analysts for wellbeing information concerning constant medical conditions, like diabetes, hepatitis and chronic drug use, has incited them to look for or legitimately acquire in any case private wellbeing records.

Fourth, the customary accentuation in scholar and strategy conversations of protection on informed assent and decision grounded in individual opportunity, can disregard the manners by which wellbeing differences and social orders' underlying shameful acts add to chronic weakness, oblige decision and lessen an open door (Skinner-Thompson, 2021; Obasagie and Darnovsky 2018; Shepherd and Wilson 2018; Scaffolds 2017). Besides, the ascent of large information and computerized reasoning in the advanced economy have made it progressively hard for any person to practice significant command over the assortment, control and utilization of restoratively related and other individual data about them (Kasperbauer 2020; Velez, 2020; Allen 2016; Cato et al. 2016; van der Sloot 2017).

1.1 Classification

"Protection" in medication frequently signifies the classification of patient-supplier experiences (counting the very reality that an experience has occurred), alongside the mystery and security of data memorialized in physical, computerized, electronic and realistic records made as a result of patient-supplier experiences (DeCew 2000; Parent 1983). Secrecy is characterized as confining data to people having a place with a bunch of explicitly approved beneficiaries (Allen 1997; Kenny 1982). Classification can be accomplished through proficient quietness and secure information the executives (Sharpe 2005; Baer et al. 2002). Thus

Sissela Bok portrayed privacy as alluding "to the limits encompassing shared privileged insights and to the most common way of monitoring these limits" (Bok 1982: 119).

Thinkers have recommended better approaches for conceptualizing natural protection and classification issues, driving the subject of security and medication into more unfamiliar headings or novel edges. For instance, it has been recommended that security and privacy in clinical practice shun the conventional basic of individual patient independence for a social comprehension that invites families and encouraging groups of people into a private circle with patients and guardians (Mohapatra and Wiley 2020). It has been suggested that conventional doctor patient privacy regulations ought to be perceived to force possibly undesirable mystery onto doctors, who bear weights of quietness they could rather not bear yet are in that frame of mind to bear by lawful responsibility to do as such (Allen, 2011).

Savants will generally concur that wellbeing is an essential part of human thriving (Faden et al. 2013; Moore 2005; Rössler 2004; Rosenberg 2000; Schoeman 1984; Boone 1983). Maimonides kept up with that substantial wellbeing is among the means and finishes of a decent life (Weiss 1991). Current thinkers by and large hold that an equitable society will be focused on getting the material and political bases of general wellbeing (Powers and Faden 2008). Logicians of medication, ethicists and bioethicists will generally concur that, with a small bunch of special cases, regarding patient secrecy benefits both individual and general wellbeing (Kamoie and Hodge 2004). They protect the act of secrecy by assorted requests to utility, nobility and prudence (Easter et al. 2004).

Expanding on the fifth century BCE Hippocratic custom of clinical parental figure mystery, western logicians protect privacy on a few utilitarian or other consequentialist grounds (Frey 2000; Bunny 1993; Freedman 1978). They contend that preventive medication, early conclusion and treatment set aside human lives and cash. People will be more disposed to certainly stand out assuming that they accept they can do so secretly. Strategy specialists keep up with that the expense of medical services and protection would be extensively higher assuming individuals stayed away from standard check-ups and brief clinical consideration since secrecy was not soundly guaranteed (Fairchild et al. 2007a). Secrecy rehearses are accepted to advance both looking for care and straight to the point exposures of wellbeing worries with regards to mind. Side effects of ailment and decline, like incontinence, cognitive decline, or pipedreams can be humiliating to discuss, even with thoughtful expert clinicians. Furthermore, commitments of secrecy can make people more able to take part in wellbeing research (Official Commission 2012; Easter et al. 2004).

Clinical classification advances the singular's clinical independence, by shielding those looking for ethically disputable clinical consideration from outside analysis and obstruction with choices (Dworkin et al. 2007; Englehardt 2000a; Feinberg 1983). Patients looking for corrective, early termination or richness medicines probably won't wish others to know their arrangements. Individuals from the overall population have now and again endeavored to impact decisions outsiders make connecting with the consideration of incapacitated newborn children, senseless or cerebrum dead family, and fetus removals. Companions, accomplices, guardians and kin have looked for contribution, with ostensibly more noteworthy moral warrant. H.J. McCloskey proposed that caring individual connections call for common responsibility (McCloskey 1971). Obviously some medical issues — grim corpulence, scoliosis, psoriasis, loss of motion — basically can't be covered from lingerie. Bioethicists, steady with general wellbeing contemplations and regulations, usually contend that secret infectious circumstances or openings ought not be hidden from weak partners and in outrageous cases could legitimize non-willful disconnection or general wellbeing quarantine (Official Commission 2015a).

Scholars have additionally offered deontological justification for safeguarding enlightening security (Penetrate 2018; Benn 1988). Hundreds of years of philosophical idea portray individuals as weak bodies and mindful spirits (Lackoff and Johnson 1999). Instructive security advances regard for human nobility, scholars has said. Parental figures show worry for moral people with normal interests and sensations of their own when they keep data about their wellbeing and wellbeing needs private (Freedman 1978).

People worried about segregation, disgrace or shame have an interest in controlling the progression of data about their wellbeing, and apparently the ethical right to do as such. Mental and other conduct medical services buyers keep on confronting shame and separation in a world in which getting what they need requires a virtual acquiescence of classification to a flock of others, including relatives, specialists, social laborers, educators, emergency clinics, back up plans, and policing (2002; AAMFT 2001; Dickson 1998).

Thoughts of moral reasonableness play into contentions for classification. Classification is seemingly expected by fair relations with government and organizations (Working environment Reasonableness, 2009, Other Web Assets). Since "information is power", exceptional worries have been brought about the way up in which government gathers and oversees individual clinical data. Unavoidable goals of fair data rehearses expect that individual information gathered about people be restricted, exact, secure and uncovered to outsiders just with assent. A few patients accept they own data about themselves, and that is all there is to it quite reasonable that they, not others, control its delivery (McGuire 2019). They might accept they own clinical data since they have bought clinical benefits (Martin 1981: 624-25). Or on the other hand they might accept they own clinical data, particularly hereditary data, since it uncovers data of a profoundly private and extraordinary sort (Laurie 2002; Rothstein 1997).

Scholars have recognized obligations of government assistance advancement, care, nobility and decency to help the case for security and privacy (Schoeman 1984). Prudence morals propose its own arrangement of justification for educational protection in medical services (van der Sloot 2017). Jennifer Radden has contended that the unique weakness of emotional wellness patients and the shame connected to their concerns transforms secrecy into a specific brand of greatness for psychological well-being care experts (Radden 2004). She has contended that the interest for secrecy in mental medication is deficiently represented on hypotheses that neglect to consider the ideals of trust and save that are signs of emotional well-being care. Ari Ezra Waldman has likewise guarded trust as a basic goodness for grasping the standardizing grounds of instructive securities. (Waldman 2018)

With regards to wellbeing research, morals advisory groups and institutional audit sheets force moral commitments on scientists to safeguard the classification of examination subjects and their clinical data (Fisher 2006; Hiatt 2003; IOM 2000).

The commitment of privacy might require the utilization of "identifiers" instead of names or "de-ID" methodology like information conglomeration (Official Commission 2012). Scientists might have to distribute genomic information in manners determined to cloud the personalities of entire families. Patient classification can be compromised in the setting of clinical talks and ground adjusts, and in the distribution and filing of clinical talks, academic articles and individual papers. Whether or not there are security concerns when just measurable use is made of people's wellbeing information has emerged. It has been contended that people have an interest in the purposes to which informational collections that incorporate their information is put, regardless of whether they are not by and by recognized by scientists (Newcombe 1994).

Security scholars alert that hardship of protection can add up to subjection, treachery and savagery

(Skinner-Thompson 2020; Gandy 1993). Most security scholars center on the damages that come from attacking the protection individual's esteem. Scholars have started additionally to think about the damages that originate from deliberate self-exposure (Allen 2011). People unreservedly unveil clinical and other touchy data about themselves. They do it in distributed journals, in virtual entertainment postings and in discussions committed to diseases, operations, physician endorsed meds, and elective medication. Ladies have webcast labor and mastectomy, referring to general wellbeing instruction objectives (Allen 2000).

Protection isn't safeguarded as a flat out great (Hixson 1987; Boone 1983; Louch 1982; Pennock and Chapman 1971; Negley 1966). Classification, for instance, is only sometimes depicted as an outright decent in medical services (Bok 1982). Savants reasonably prescribe significant exemptions for the act of secrecy. In the first place, all medical care suppliers and capable grown-ups ought to be committed to report proof of misuse or disregard of minor youngsters, like unexplained cracks and unhealthiness, regardless of whether the security interests of the kids and additionally their victimizers would appear to recommend in any case (Dickson 1998). Disappointment of clinical laborers to speedily unveil can have destructive ramifications for weak minors. While classification choices are passed on to people or their watchmen in many occasions, minor kids are a solid exemption because of their lacking mental and moral limits and because of the likelihood that their gatekeepers are victimizers who might profit from privacy. Second, cherished in American regulation as the Tarasoff Rule, emotional well-being suppliers have a moral obligation to caution police or likely casualties of deranged patients' fierce impending goals (Doors and Arons 1999). These two special cases mirror a conviction that keeping away from actual injury to outsiders is a higher priority than perpetually conceding to patients' inclinations, saving their sentiments and safeguarding their confidence in connections. Significant philosophical inquiries emerge about the degree of "Good Samaritan" obligations, whistle-blowing commitments and the obligation to caution in medical care settings. Crediting such obligations possibly encroaches the freedom people in any case appreciate to act and cease from going about as they see fit inasmuch as they don't certifiably hurt others. Ostensibly the individual who declines to help or caution isn't the mindful reason for the maltreatment and viciousness that occurs for other people. However helpfulness contends for okay, minimal expense intercessions to forestall serious damage.

Third, there might be circumstances in which clinical secrecy ought not to be safeguarded on the grounds that the general population has an option to be aware. One class of data which people in general or general wellbeing authorities are normally remembered to reserve an option to know is data about examples of profoundly irresistible infectious sicknesses with high paces of mortality and dreariness, like ebola, Coronavirus, HIV/Helps, hepatitis and measles. One more class of data considered not reasonable for secrecy is data the media has a privilege to distribute as an issue of its newsworthiness. Emotional clinical salvages of auto collision casualties are naturally newsworthy occasions. It has been contended that the general population has an option to be familiar with public authorities' serious clinical issues; maybe more than specialists have commonly revealed (Robins and Rothschild 1988; Thompson 1987). In the US, offended parties in private injury claims are approached to submit to clinical assessment; and attorneys and fantastic juries have the power to summon clinical data for use in judicial actions and examinations, setting exceptionally delicate clinical data in danger of public revelation (Wolf and Zandecki 2006). Like the requests of general wellbeing observation, lawful cycle requests contend against unfit privileges of clinical classification (El Emam and Moher 2013).

1.2 Mystery

Sissela Bok characterized mystery as deliberate covering (Bok 1982). Patients and parental figures can advance protection through mystery. Mystery rehearses pose a potential threat in medical services. Certain individuals don't share the information on clinical side effects even with their dearest companions and relatives. An individual may subtly know the person is sick before the individual in question lets it out to relatives or counsels a doctor. Hesitance to impart information on clinical side effects to partners or family and clinical experts might come from dread of handicap or demise; evasion of separation in protection, work and schooling; or fear of social disgrace, disgrace, humiliation or dismissal. During the 1990s, questions emerged about the commitments of dental specialists and other medical services suppliers to forgo mystery and uncover their HIV positive status to patients. Ripeness patients might need to hide the utilization of given sperm or eggs, because of the social and strict results of revelation (Birenbaum-Carmeli et al. 2008). Not many ailments or strategies are covered in absolute mystery any longer. However, individuals might like to maintain mystery the reality of, for instance, their elective corrective techniques, weight reduction medical procedure, sex reassignment medical procedure, early terminations, ripeness therapies, and sanitizations.

Paternalistically keeping clinical information from patients as the mysteries of specialists, sound mates and grown-up youngsters sets beliefs of usefulness in providing care in opposition to the patient's more right than wrong to be aware. Paternalistic mystery is a significant component of clinical practice, more predominant in certain nations, networks and families than others. Moral standards of independence and organization contend for illuminating patients regarding their ailments, honestly and completely. However, clinical news is once in a while purposely kept from patients.

There is no assurance that patients will accept clinical insights or determinations solidly positioned before them by qualified doctors. Disavowal of unsavory bits of insight is ordinary. Self-trickery about wellbeing is a strong peculiarity. Certain individuals earnestly think that declining to acknowledge an undesirable determination by keeping an inspirational perspective will protect them from clinical disaster. Mental problems can fool one into thinking one is well, cheerful and shrewd, as opposed to the hyper, fanciful individual the specialist might analyze.

One more sort of mystery rehearsed in medication is the disguise of careful injuries and scars. Restorative specialists conceal scars inside hairlines and in the wrinkles behind the ears. Bosom malignant growth is at this point not the reason for mystery it used to be, yet recreation medical procedure following mastectomy is a sort of covering. The bait of negligibly intrusive laparoscopic medical procedure isn't just that it might both diminish the length of clinic stays and the gamble of disease, yet additionally that it leaves less conspicuous and apparent scars. Progresses in clinical envisioning, for example, the X-beam, X-ray, CT sweep and ultrasound, permit suppliers to enter the body and catch data without leaving indications of having done as such.

Neuroimaging, mind envisioning innovations (Touch) for the most part, and high level falsehood location bring up basic issues about whether secret contemplations ought to be accessible for acumen, and provided that this is true under what conditions (Official Commission 2014; Farahany 2012). The issue is one of pressured self-revelation and, in the event that some time or another criminal responsibility could be dependably perceived from imaging, self-implication.

1.3 Information Assurance and Security

The ethical importance joined to clinical protection is reflected in information assurance and security regulations embraced by neighborhood and public specialists all over the planet. The mark of these regulations is to direct the assortment, quality, putting away, sharing and maintenance of wellbeing information, including the electronic wellbeing record (EHR) (CDT 2009, in Other Web Assets). Wellbeing protection rules limit revelation without even a trace of informed assent; however common resolutions perceive various special cases for routine purposes, research, general wellbeing revealing, and legitimate interaction and policing. The approach agreement is by all accounts that, while clinical protection is significant, patients' clinical data might be revealed to outsiders for socially significant purposes irrelevant to their own consideration. Electronically put away and delivered clinical data is by its very nature portable. Those with access can communicate EHR information across town or across state and public boundaries. Patients today have extraordinary admittance to their own wellbeing data. Patients might send clinical information over email, share it with outsider cloud information capacity suppliers, or gather wellbeing information through applications and wearable gadgets with little thoughtfulness regarding third part access and use.

A few wards have extraordinary standards for the executives of specific wellbeing data. Information with respect to HIV/Helps, emotional well-being and hereditary qualities are managed the cost of exceptional treatment in U.S. regulation, for instance. Logicians consider whether specific circumstances legitimacy such superiority. The contention for HIV/Helps superiority reviews the beginning of the worldwide plague when information on the sickness was poor, therapy was ineffectual, and social disgrace connected to burden. The contention for emotional wellness excellence is that patients do and should "uncovered their spirits" to mental and conduct wellbeing suppliers, making exposures socially exorbitant (Radden 2004). A U.S. government rule precludes basing business or medical coverage choices on data about an individual's DNA or hereditary inclinations (GINA 2008). The main contention for hereditary information excellence has all the earmarks of being that hereditary information passes on interestingly itemized data about an individual and her natural family, data an individual could reserve a privilege to be aware or a right not to be aware (Chadwick et al. 2014). Some hereditary data can predict an individual's wellbeing future (Laurie 2002; Rothstein 1997).

The utilization of electronic innovation has been depicted as an aid for medical services conveyance and organization for quite a long time (Burton 2004; Public Exploration Gathering 1991). However uplifted worries for protection followed expanded compactness of wellbeing information commanded by regulation (HIPAA 1996) and outsider ("cloud") information capacity. The commitment to safeguard clinical information held by the state or privately owned businesses has taken on criticalness as increasingly more wellbeing information is being sent and put away electronically. It has been contended that data chiefs owe it to general society to go to severe lengths to forestall information breaks and to fittingly answer and remediate when a break happens. An information break can result from the robbery of a PC; false or coincidental admittance to information; damage by exploitative or disappointed workers; or the deficiency of information stockpiling gadgets. Significant medical clinics, wellbeing organizations and guarantors have encountered exceptionally plugged information breaks influencing a great many customers whose names, addresses, wellbeing recognizable proof numbers and different information were compromised (Seh et al. 2020). A philosophical inquiry raised by information breaks is the manner by which to characterize and ethically fix hurt. Clinical data fraud and public revelation of private realities are for the most part viewed as "hurts" (Biegelman 2009). However, it has been contended that carelessly causing expanded dangers of data fraud and public revelation of private realities are hurts, as well. In the event that risk enhancement is hurt, however, it hazy ought to consider fair remuneration or moral fix.

1.4 Obscurity

Obscurity has esteem in an assortment of general wellbeing and clinical examination settings. Research distributions normally safeguard the personalities of biomedical examination subjects or clinical patients. Exceptional consideration is paid to hereditary data. Albeit various unmistakable researchers and laypeople have disclosed their genomes, hereditary qualities research and academic distribution norms call for insurance of the characters of exploration subjects and their families. Bioethicists recognize recognizable, de-distinguished and anonymized entire genome sequencing information. (Official Commission, 2012) In the US, de-recognized information isn't safeguarded under the regulations safeguarding human subjects known as the Normal Rule. Concerns can emerge about whether specific techniques for de-recognizable proof and anonymization enough safeguard people from attack of protection and breaks of secrecy (Yoo et al. 2018). "Differential protection" is an anonymization way to deal with individual information sharing inclined toward by PC researchers that has likely worth to medical services information (Dwork 2006).

The utilization of the secretly conveyed individual journal for finding out about and evaluating wellbeing related conduct is typical (Minichiello et al. 2000). Research subjects are approached to record contraception use, condom use and other sexual practices in journals which become research devices. Analysts should accept care to caution research subjects about the risks of uncovering data which could open them to social or lawful approvals.

With regards to Coronavirus, North American arrangement creators were given individuals from the public who hid their contaminated status and decided to go on planes, gather and not wear veils. In the prime of the HIV/Helps emergency in North America, policymakers correspondingly battled to find morally sound ways to deal with irresistible infectious prevention despite defective consistence with suggested accepted procedures. Contention emerged during the 1990s over mysterious testing. Unknown HIV/Helps testing is currently regularly performed however was once dubious among ethicists. Secrecy was shielded on the ground that it empowered testing by people wishing to control when, whether and to whom to unveil their HIV/Helps status (Fairchild et al. 2007a). Then again, it was perceived that social reconnaissance is a possibly helpful part of forcefully safeguarding general wellbeing (Fairchild et al. 2007b; Gallagher et al. 2007; Burr 1999); in certain circumstances, unknown testing could make following examples of disease more troublesome. It was recommended that unknown testing permitted tainted people to participate in hazardous, ethically flippant sexual way of behaving without responsibility. Advocates of mysterious testing answered that strategy producers and ethicists shouldn't accept that people who learn they are HIV positive based on unknown tests would selfishly hide their status from sexual accomplices. A couple of people will intentionally force serious dangers on others, however recently educated positive test-takers may mindfully inform past and future accomplices, cease from hazardous ways of behaving, and look for clinical consideration. The moral issues encompassing HIV/Helps have changed now that the condition is less disparaging and, in created nations, is a treatable constant condition as opposed to a capital punishment.

1.5 Responsibility

Privacy flourishes as a lawful obligation and institutional practice, in spite of the rising pattern towards deliberate receptiveness about private clinical data. The points of interest of wellbeing and clinical consideration have become adequate subjects of conventional discussion outside the family circle. In the U.S., well known people have started to lead the pack, standing in opposition to their Coronavirus, respiratory failures, Helps, erectile brokenness, dementia, Parkinson's sickness, melanoma, prostate disease and bosom malignant growth. Many would have thought of Divulgences that as indelicate or demonizing quite a while back are made unreservedly today, whether to make discussion, share a worry, instruct the general population, or underwrite a non-benefit or drug item.

To an important degree, transparency is likewise constrained by ethics and regulation. Responsibility for individual life is an element of current life, and clinical responsibility is a component of present day life. Being responsible means being called upon to share data make sense of, change conduct or submit to endorse. Right after Coronavirus, SARS, Ebola and Helps, new degrees of data responsibility acquired public acknowledgment. Around the world, individuals are coming to consider minor and major infectious sicknesses conditions bringing about open responsibility. The responsibility that is called for incorporates data assembling and sharing as a state of movement among urban communities and nations or entering working environments and schools. Worldwide explorers are approached to report side effects of ailment to authorities. Global guests have their internal heat levels examined for fever consequently as they continue to customs in certain air terminals, laborers are requested equivalent to a condition from enters work environments. Compulsory testing, detailing, contact following and the utilization of endorsed side effect checking applications, are instances of wellbeing data responsibility. Past responsibility for wellbeing data, the Coronavirus pandemic has made individuals responsible for cover wearing, hand washing, self-confinement, party and different ways of behaving once thought to be simply private. Choices whether to immunize are likewise dependent upon moral and legitimate responsibility, whether to forestall measles, Coronavirus, or influenza.

Many individuals talk transparently about wellbeing matters with outsiders as a state of getting and paying for medical services. For instance, a family requiring the help of a provincial psychological wellness/mental impediment organization undeniably puts reams of delicate data in the possession of government. (Spans 2017) The equivalent is valid for a family which necessities to apply for government benefits for maturing or handicapped kinfolk. The more divulgences a family should make, the more extensive the circle of secrecy and the lesser the clinical protection. Inquiries of distributive equity are raised by required divulgences to government made as a state of admittance to mind. Poor and crippled people subject to clinical help from government have significantly less enlightening protection opposite government than rich and sound people. The dangers and weights of state information on the individual are lopsidedly borne by the un-well off sections of society.

1.6 Expert Standards

The obligation of secrecy is a center agreement standard inside medical care (Currie 2005). One significant appearance of this agreement in the U.S. has been the advancement of the "declaration of privacy" by which analysts announce that secrecy is of particular interest to their subjects (Wolf and Zandecki 2006, Wolf et al. 2004). The mechanical age has led to the call for medical care suppliers, even the people who work alone or in little gatherings, to be forceful in the reception of capable data rehearse. Everything would concur that office practices would be able and ought to be intended to safeguard the character of clients and the protection of discussions. Normal understandings are that specialists ought to be prudent in the assortment of data; they ought to store treatment notes and keeps in a safe way; they ought to share data just with assent or as legally necessary; and they ought to safeguard delicate data in it's on the web and disconnected structures utilizing locks, passwords, encryption and other fitting gadgets. Delicate data that is not generally required ought not to be held endlessly.

Medical services suppliers are attributed moral commitments to try not to nonchalantly talk about classified patient matters in online entertainment or in email that may not be completely private or secure (Chretien et al. 2011). They should try not to talk about quiet matters on cell phones in broad daylight places, for example, in office passageways, emergency clinic entryways and on trains. Classification can be abused by unapproved accounts and divulgence of clinical photos. Photography assumes a part in clinical specializations including dermatology and plastic medical procedure, giving raise to worries about moral purposes of realistic pictures of patients' countenances and bodies. At the very least educated agree would give off an impression of being expected for making and unveiling photos on whose premise an individual could be recognized. Morally basic assent was not gotten in a famous U.S. case: it became known in 2013 that a doctor partnered with Johns Hopkins College Clinic subtly recorded many his obstetrics and gynecology patients with explicit aim (Allen 2015). Recording has come to assume a standard part in family treatment and isn't viewed as dishonest by common experts (AAMFT 2001). Numerous clinicians trust the restorative and preparing advantages of recording offset the dangers of unapproved use or divulgence. Regardless of whether unapproved use or exposure was not a worry, a moral inquiry would remain. Should conduct wellbeing clients be called upon to make accounts which intrinsically penance the protection of their homes, interchanges and articulations of feelings?

Doctors are discussing whether to build the utilization of video and sound taping in routine clinical practice, medical procedure and exploration, and bioethicists are showing up (Blaauw et al. 2014; Makary 2013). Should office visits be recorded as a feature of the standard clinical record? From one perspective, accounts would resolve the issue of defective memory and fragmented experience notes. Accounts could record informed assent systems and give proof to deflect or uphold negligence suits. Then again, accounts could hinder patients and increment their distress. Recording practices could urge doctors to be less mindful of the patients before them on the hypothesis that they can constantly "return to the tape" for subtleties.

2. Actual Security

There has been somewhat little consideration paid by savants to actual security worries in medication contrasted with educational worries. However normal patients bring flock serious areas of strength for of humility, isolation and substantial respectability to specialists' workplaces, clinics, telemedicine visits and other medical care experiences. These assumptions that they won't be unnecessarily contacted, swarmed, gaped at or furtively shot, recorded or imaged connect with the requirement for mental solace, nobility and security. The web has made conveying medical care conceivable across tremendous distances. (Chepesiuk 1999). Telemedicine, which developed dramatically during the principal year if the Coronavirus emergency, permitted specialists and attendants to assess normal clinical grievances from a distance without contacting the patient. Meanwhile, medical care commonly includes actual contact with others.

2.1 Isolation

Isolation is a type of actual protection of unique interest to clinical morals (Storr 2005; Barbour 2004). The wiped out don't have any desire to be forlorn and deserted; however they might need individual existence alone. Isolation has esteem as a setting for calm reflection about the meaning of sickness and injury. A time of isolation after conference and self-training is a helpful condition wherein to decide on treatment choices.

The most diseased patients may both long for and dread isolation. At the point when alone they encounter the possibly savage truth of looming demise. However in organization they might feel disparaged or remorseful about the weights they force on loved ones. Whether the enduring is the misery of injury, labor, recuperating from significant medical procedure or biting the dust, people might feel that they shouldn't need to manage others while in such a state or at such a period. Certain accepted practices approve conceding to wishes of the debilitated or biting the dust for disengagement and isolation (Post 1989; Nissenbaum 2009). These desires might emerge and be disregarded not just in medical clinic, hospice or nursing home settings, yet in addition in mental medical clinics and detainment facilities, where panoptic strategies of checking and observation win (Bozovic 1995; Holmes and Federman 2006: 16-17; Foucault 1977).

2.2 Substantial Humility

Scholars in the ideals morals and Christian morals customs have distinguished humility as an ethical uprightness (Schueler 1999). Humility is a type of actual security of extraordinary interest to clinical morals. Assuming patients are to get the best consideration, they should open their bodies to clinical staff and specialists. Taking off one's clothing for reasons for assessment and testing is standard for most medical care customers. Occupied trauma centers and neighborhood facilities might not be able to shroud or detach patients by any stretch of the imagination. Harried doctors might neglect "bedside habits" and flop adequately to respect patients' humility assumptions. In-patients in showing clinics are supposed to adjust to reduced actual security, since clinical understudies and analysts go with going to doctors on adjusts and partake in care.

Made in the USA
Columbia, SC
23 February 2023

12874578R00085